# Scripting

## A Guide for Nurses

Kathleen L. Garrison, MSN, RN
Jo-Ann C. Byrne, RN, BS, MHSA
Frances Moore, RNC, BSN, MSA

## ⊢HCPro

*Quick-E! Pro Scripting: A Guide for Nurses* is published by HCPro, Inc.

HCPro, Inc., provides information resources for the healthcare industry.

HCPro, Inc., is not affiliated in any way with The Joint Commission, which owns the JCAHO and Joint Commission trademarks. MAGNET™, MAGNET RECOGNITION PROGRAM®, and ANCC MAGNET RECOGNITION® are trademarks of the American Nurses Credentialing Center (ANCC). The products and services of HCPro, Inc., and The Greeley Company are neither sponsored nor endorsed by the ANCC. The acronym MRP is not a trademark of HCPro or its parent corporation.

Kathleen L. Garrison, MSN, RN, Author
Jo-Ann C. Byrne, RN, BS, MHSA, Author
Frances Moore, RNC, BSN, MSA, Author
Michael Briddon, Senior Managing Editor
Emily Sheahan, Group Publisher
Mike Mirabello, Senior Graphic Artist

Adam Carroll, Copyeditor
Amy Cohen, Proofreader
Susan Darbyshire, Art Director
Matt Sharpe, Production Supervisor
Claire Cloutier, Editorial Services Manager
Jean St. Pierre, Director of Operations

Advice given is general. Readers should consult professional counsel for specific legal, ethical, or clinical questions.

Arrangements can be made for quantity discounts. For more information, contact:

HCPro, Inc.
P.O. Box 1168
Marblehead, MA 01945
Telephone: 800/650-6787 or 781/639-1872
Fax: 781/639-2982
E-mail: *customerservice@hcpro.com*

**Visit HCPro at its World Wide Web sites:**
*www.hcpro.com* and *www.hcmarketplace.com*

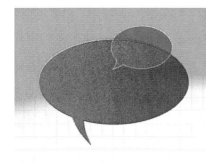

# Contents

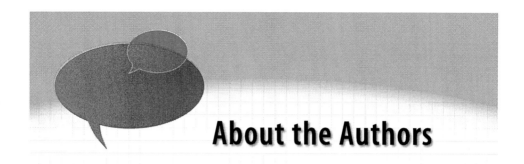

# About the Authors

## Kathleen L. Garrison, MSN, RN

**Kathleen L. Garrison, MSN, RN,** has been a registered nurse for 28 years. She graduated in 1980 with her BSN from Fairfield (CT) University and earned her master's degree in nursing in 2005 from George Mason University in Fairfax, VA.

Since beginning her nursing career, Garrison has gained expertise and served in various roles in many specialties, including burns, critical care, home health, and emergency nursing.

Garrison is the clinical educator in the training and development department at Prince William Hospital in Manassas, VA. Throughout her career at Prince William, she has progressively climbed the ladder of responsibility, from staff RN to charge nurse to clinical nurse leader, and has functioned in a variety of management roles.

Garrison lives in Manassas with her husband, Jim; three children: Emily, Kaitlin, and Jimmy; and their bichon frisé, Jingle.

## Jo-Ann C. Byrne, RN, BS, MHSA

**Jo-Ann C. Byrne, RN, BS, MHSA,** has more than 40 years of experience in healthcare. Her career began as an emergency department nurse and critical care educator. She has worked as a nurse, nurse manager, educator, and director of education in a variety of hospital settings.

Byrne is a former lieutenant in the U.S. Navy Nurse Corps and has held senior management and consultant positions at Booz Allen Hamilton and Deloitte Consulting Group.

Byrne is currently the director of education and organizational development at St. Vincent's Healthcare in Jacksonville, FL, where she oversees all education, training development, and implementation activities for the hospital system.

In June 2006, Byrne coauthored the book *The Successful Leadership Development Program: How to Build It and How to Keep It Going.*

## Frances Moore, RNC, BSN, MSA

**Frances Moore, RNC, BSN, MSA,** is a nurse manager and clinical educator with more than 30 years of experience in healthcare. She has mentored many nurses as they develop their leadership skills in running a nursing unit and has set an example as an excellent clinician in neonatal ICU and mother-baby units.

Moore currently serves as manager of the department of education and organizational development at St. Vincent's Healthcare in Jacksonville, FL. She leads the education team for a two-hospital health system and is responsible for a variety of educational opportunities.

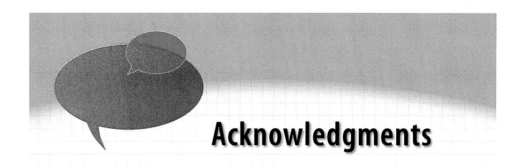

# Acknowledgments

## Kathleen L. Garrison, MSN, RN

It takes a special person to be a nurse. It does not matter what we specialize in; we are all special. In my nearly 30 years of nursing, I have met so many professionals who have unknowingly given a part of themselves to me. My portion of this book is dedicated to them. From my humble beginnings as a new graduate in the burn unit to my experiences in home health as a physician office nurse, as an ER nurse, and from my current peers and mentors in staff development and education, you have taught me a lot and it has been a pleasure to work alongside you. Wherever you are today, thank you.

Thanks also go out to my loving family. Without you, there is no purpose in my life. "Love you all more!"

And thank you to Mike, our editor, for another opportunity to be creative and share with my nursing community. "Is there anything else I can do for you? I have the time!"

## Jo-Ann C. Byrne, RN, BS, MHSA

I've been a nurse for more than 40 years. Whether it was managing an ER, consulting with a client, or leading a seminar, much of the knowledge and skill I rely on today came from discipline and solid training early in my career. Those first, formative years after nursing school were spent in the Navy Nurse Corps. The men and women with whom I served were some of the best in the world. My portion of this book is dedicated to them and those who continue to serve us today. I am eternally grateful.

To my family, much love. To my Papa, I miss you.

I owe the pleasure of this experience to Mike, our editor. Thank you for the opportunity. I look forward to more!

## Frances Moore, RNC, BSN, MSA

First, I would like to thank Jo-Ann for offering me the opportunity to participate in creating this book with her. This was my first endeavor in the publishing world, and it has been a wonderful experience to work with dedicated nursing professionals like her and Kathy. It has been an exciting adventure, and I am ready to try it again!

To Mike, our editor, for your guidance: You make it look so easy!

Thank you to my wonderful husband and parents for their support, guidance, and encouragement throughout the years!

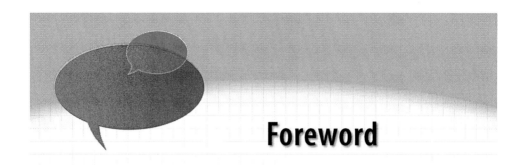

# Foreword

## It Is Time for Our Profession to Embrace Scripting

*by Shelley Cohen, RN, BS, CEN*

The nursing profession is constantly changing the way it delivers healthcare. On a daily basis, nurses assess, diagnose, plan, intervene, and evaluate outcomes of our patients. As our experiences and knowledge base grow and develop, new methods and models of care emerge that enhance our current practices. Going back to foundation principles, it is this very nursing theory that drives all we do for our patients.

Of the many tools nurses use to be effective, communication is clearly an essential one. It plays an integral role in our delivery of patient care. As a profession, nursing needs to embrace the concept of scripting as a way to enhance how we communicate.

Simply put, it is the prudent nurse that will recognize the value of scripting and embrace its acceptance in healthcare communication. Whether it is feeling better prepared prior to meeting with an angry family member or bringing confidence into your phone conversation with a provider, scripting is empowering. And with customer satisfaction remaining as a constant indicator of quality care, guided comments and responses shift patient and family perceptions. In appreciating the positive effect scripting has had in venues outside of healthcare, such as aviation and other customer service programs, it is time for nursing to recognize its value.

Scripting affects consistency in practice and is not only related to how we perform tasks and procedures—it is also associated with how we communicate to the patient or family prior to carrying out these interventions. As we know, poor communication has been proven to lead to errors and risk within patient care.

Many nurses and nurse leaders do not understand the premise of scripting and have been incorrectly taught that it is about memorizing a statement. By providing an alternative method of communication, scripting empowers the nurse with options to respond to challenging or potentially risky scenarios. It's clear that we need autonomy in the profession, and we want to encourage nurses to use their positive attributes as they work with patients.

Let's take a look at two quick examples where scripting can be effective. The first example involves staff members who demonstrate unacceptable behaviors; nurse managers are often challenged by this situation. Despite warnings and threats of disciplinary action, the nurse leader may sometimes feel as though staff members are not listening. The use of scripting allows the manager to proactively prepare responses that demonstrate expectations and place accountability where it belongs. For example:

- **Common response:** "I am sorry you were late again and have to be placed on a second-level warning."

- **Scripted response:** "It is unfortunate you opted to be late again today. You are now on a second-level warning. My expectation is that you will not be late again this time period. If you are, you will be required to take a day off without pay while being placed on a third-level warning. Do you have any questions?"

See the difference? Instead of simply providing a general, punitive reaction, the scripted response demonstrated expectations and called for accountability.

The second example involves staff members dealing with coworkers, patients, or families who are uncooperative or have unrealistic expectations. Left to communicate on their own, staff members struggle to find the right words or, at times, exacerbate the situation by using the wrong ones. For example:

- **Common scenario:** "Mary, I am running out for a quick smoke break. Will you watch my people?"

- **Common response:** "Sure. I guess."

- **Scripted responses:** "I can't, Mary. I have three procedures to do. You will need to find someone else," or, "I am actually taking a break right now, so I can't."

These scripted responses—and the collection of examples in the pages of this valuable resource—help us to demonstrate empathy and an understanding of the needs of our patients, families, and coworkers. By providing tools and resources that enhance our communication, we improve patient care and make our work environments healthier. And those goals, regardless of the enhancements and developments within healthcare, will never change.

# Reacquaint Yourself with Scripting

Scripting is a tool. It is designed to give you, the nurse, guidelines for handling given situations more effectively.

Scripting is almost as old as nursing. Think back to your first few weeks of Nursing 101. Do you remember that first bed bath? Every step was laid out—scripted—for you: what you would do, what you would observe, what you would report as a result of your observations. All of it was to assist you in picking up subtle changes in your patient's status. When you learned to administer medications, you learned the "Five Rights." This script helped to decrease the chance that you would make a medication error.

So, as you can see, scripting isn't new.

During the past 10 years, we have been hearing and reading much more about scripting in journals, at professional conferences, and on the Internet. The concept is definitely not without its controversy.

The service industry became enamored with scripting many years ago. Just look at franchises such as McDonald's, Burger King, and Starbucks. Hotels are another big scripting industry. Staff members say "My pleasure" and "Is there anything else I can do for you?" hundreds of times on a daily basis.

Healthcare officially started scripting in housekeeping (environmental services) to improve customer satisfaction scores. Cue cards like the example in Figure 1 were handed out, and training sessions were held to instruct staff members on the attitude, tone of voice, and demeanor that should accompany the words.

---

**Figure 1**　　　　　　　　　　　　　　　　　　　　　　　**Cue card example**

**Entering room:**
Good morning. I'm _____, and I am here to clean your room.
Is there anything special you would like me to do?
I want to provide you excellent service.

**Leaving room:**
I'm finished cleaning your room. If any housekeeping issues come up, just call the number (8000) on this card (hold up tent card). I hope I have provided you with excellent service.

**End with one of these:**
God bless you./I'll keep you in my prayers (if appropriate).
I'll keep you in my thoughts. I hope today goes well for you.

---

The majority of these initiatives were driven by customer and patient satisfaction scores. As patient satisfaction scores began to take center stage, scripting spread to other areas of our organizations, such as telephone operators, registration staff members, and nursing. This book will focus on the nursing angle and show how scripting can be used in a variety of scenarios and situations.

 **Quick Highlight:** Throughout, be on the lookout for "quick highlights" that will drive home some of the most crucial points in the book.

In the next eight chapters, we'll explore how scripting can help you in your daily interactions with peers, physicians, and patients. And we'll show how it can be empowering.

First, though, let's take a look at the controversial side of scripting and the value it can bring to your nursing life.

　　　　　　　　　　　　　　　　　　**Quick-E! Pro: Scripting**

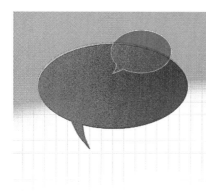

# CHAPTER 1

# The Value of Scripting

## Learning Objectives

After reading this chapter, you will be able to:

- Define scripting

- Identify two communication models often used in nursing

- List the components of SBAR

> "The exchange may feel unnatural, even awkward. But scripted talk is more than just an annoying quirk of the modern service economy. It represents a deep form of managerial control—a regimentation of the labor process so total that it extends even to speech."
>
> —Adria Scharf, as quoted in *Dollars & Sense: The Magazine of Economic Justice.*

Although this is only one person's opinion, the perspective is unfortunately shared by many.

Nursing unions picked up the perspective and a headline in the April 2006 *Massachusetts Nurse Newsletter* read, "Newton-Wellesley RNs Oppose Wal-Martinization of Nursing Practice." The article went on to say, "We are NOT Stepford RNs. As professional nurses, how we communicate with our patients and what we say to them is our professional prerogative based on the needs of the patient and the preservation of an appropriate therapeutic relationship" (Massachusetts Nurses Association).

A third opinion states, "Nurses are now mandated to script to patients ... they want to convince people that it will reduce falls and injuries. Safe staffing will reduce falls and injuries!" (Safestaffing.info). Although staffing levels have been discussed from California to New York for a very long time, scripting has never been suggested as a solution to safe staffing.

Scripting *is* used to help nurses communicate important information to patients and to calm patients' fears. Controversial, yes, but when implemented and practiced, scripting is a very valuable tool.

Furthermore, research has shown that scripting dramatically increases the patient's perception of delivered care quality (Ryan and Wojiciechowski 2003). Florida's Winter Haven Hospital provides a more specific example. After using scripting in the radiology department for only 60 days in 2006, a survey revealed that quality of care scores increased by 2%, obtaining results scores jumped by 10%, and recommended to return scores increased by 9% (*Radiology Management* 2007).

## So what exactly is scripting?

*Merriam-Webster*'s defines scripting as:

1. To prepare a script for or from

2. To provide carefully considered details for (as a plan of action)

This is exactly what scripting is used for: to be sure we have a *plan*. Not just any plan, but a plan of action that will, to the best of our ability, ensure that patients have good experiences and positive outcomes.

In *The Patient Access Director's Handbook,* Wolfskill and Lipka write, "Scripting involves identifying common situations, activities, and questions ... and teaching staff how to answer appropriately to project the caring, professional image of a staff member" (Wolfskill and Lipka 2008). They go on to say that the most difficult part of the process is developing the responses.

## A quick look at communication models

In nursing across the country, you will find a multitude of communication models. Some models have been homegrown and work very well; others have been developed, written about, and marketed with great success. One model developed by the Studer Group that is often mentioned is AIDET (acknowledge, introduce, duration, explanation, and thank you). AIDET guides the speaker through the critical elements of a conversation, which the Studer Group refers to as the "Five Fundamentals of Service." Let's take a closer look in Figure 2.

**Figure 2**                                                                                          **AIDET**

| | |
|---|---|
| Acknowledges the patient | Smile and make eye contact<br>Call the patient by his or her last name |
| Introduces self | Your name, role, and what you're going to do<br>Why you're qualified to do it |
| Duration of the task or test | Length of time: process, procedure, waiting, etc. |
| Explanation | What's next, what tools you're using, who's coming, what you're doing, and why |
| Thanks the patient | A stronger sense of involvement<br>"We're glad you chose us" |

This conversational style allows you to clearly communicate with anyone while including key pieces of information designed to specifically gain trust, increase compliance, and improve the clinical experience.

Another model that has emerged in scripting communities is SBAR (situation, background, assessment, and recommendation). Many, upon hearing the acronym, associate it with nurse-physician interactions. SBAR is widely used for this level of communication, and physicians and nurses agree it has merit. Staff members have learned that communication with physicians is more successful when the nurse has the right information before he or she makes the phone call. We'll discuss this in greater detail in Chapter 4.

More globally, SBAR can create a shared model for transfer of information regardless of the recipients, as in the following example:

- Situation: What is happening?

- Background: What circumstances led to this?

- Assessment: What do you think the problem is?

- Recommendation: What do you want to do?

Figure 3 provides two templates, one filled in and one blank, that you can use to help insert SBAR into your daily practice.

| Figure 3 | | SBAR sheet |
|---|---|---|

| **S** Situation 8–12 seconds | **This is (your name) from unit _____, and I am calling about:** _____. (List two identifiers such as patient name & DOB) **The problem I am calling about is:** (briefly state the problem—what it is, when it started, and how severe) |
|---|---|
| **B** Background Set the context for this urgent problem | **Admitted for:** _____ **Pertinent history:** _____ **Pertinent labs/test results:** _____ **Current therapy:** (pertinent meds, IVF, treatments, monitoring, etc.) _____ **Current VS:** BP ___ / ___ HR ___ RR ___ Sats ___% Temp ___ °F **Other clinical info:** |
| **A** Assessment | **This is what I think the problem is:** (assessment of what is happening) |
| **R** Recommend | **I suggest or request that you:** (say what you would like to see done) **Labs/imaging?** CXR, ABG, EKG, CBC, COAGS, cultures, BMP? **Possible consults:** _____ **Is a higher level of care needed?** Telemetry, ICU, etc. What questions do you have for me? My name is _____. I am here until _____ and can be reached at Ext. _____. |

*Source: Arizona Hospital and Healthcare Association SBAR Toolkit. Used with permission.*

| | |
|---|---|
| **Figure 3** | **SBAR sheet (cont.)** |

| | |
|---|---|
| **S**<br>*Situation*<br><br>8–12 seconds | |
| **B**<br>*Background*<br><br>Set the context for this urgent problem | |
| **A**<br>*Assessment* | |
| **R**<br>*Recommend* | What questions do you have for me? My name is _____.<br>I am here until _____ and can be reached at Ext. _____. |

*Source: Arizona Hospital and Healthcare Association SBAR Toolkit. Used with permission.*

## A note to nursing leaders

We all know that strong communication skills contribute to excellence in customer service. Consistency in communication is just as important. If you're thinking about scripting, even on a small scale to start, here are some things to keep in mind:

- Almost every patient interaction can be scripted. The more information you can provide for staff members, the more confident they will feel.

- Be consistent. Everyone needs to be saying the same things.

- Scripts serve as guides. Ensure that essential words and language are included, but let staff members develop the scripts in their own language. If the scripts feel and sound natural, staff members will use them.

- Hold training sessions to communicate the goal of scripting. Role-playing is a great way for staff members to develop a comfort level with scripts. If there are staff members who still feel a bit stiff about the process, encourage them to practice.

We should remember that, in many instances, staff members have already created scripts for themselves. Very often, those scripts do not contain the messages we want delivered. The wrong things are said to patients every day.

**Quick Highlight:** To ensure that your message is clear and consistent and to avoid potential misunderstandings, consider scripting.

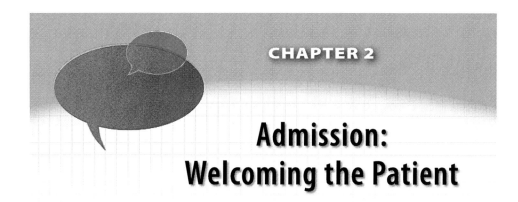

# CHAPTER 2

# Admission:
# Welcoming the Patient

## Learning Objectives

After reading this chapter you will be able to:

■ Discuss the appropriate steps to take after a patient is admitted

As a nurse, you walk into the hospital every day. You say "hi" to your colleagues, grab a drink of water, and get ready to accept your patient assignments. But what if it wasn't so familiar? What if walking through the front door of your facility was like walking into a foreign place? What if you felt lost and confused?

Every day, new patients enter into hospital hallways for the first time. It's up to you as the nurse to make them feel comfortable—and more importantly, safe. By following some simple guidelines, you can make sure the admission process goes smoothly every time.

## Simple communication goes a long way

Mrs. St. John, a 68-year-old white female, was just admitted to your unit accompanied by her husband and son. She suffered a syncopal episode at home, was seen by her family physician, and was directly admitted to your unit. Her family requested a private room, but a semi-private is currently the only one available.

As mentioned previously, whether patients are admitted routinely, unexpectedly, or urgently, each one experiences fear and concern. Using detailed scripting to give thought to the admission process prior to a patient's arrival will provide consistent and complete information each and every time.

At the outset, make sure to:

- Greet the patient by name

- Introduce yourself

- Make the acquaintance of the family

- Introduce roommate (if applicable)

Here is an example of a script for Mrs. St. John:

"Hello Mrs. St. John, I am Anne Seton. I'll be your nurse today and would like to welcome you to 4 East. Who is accompanying you today? I understand you requested a private room, but currently there are none available. We have notified the desk of your request, but in the meantime, I would like to introduce you to your roommate, Mrs. Parker. She has been with us a few days, and I am sure you and she will have lots to talk about."

Do you remember the first time you were a patient? Anxiety is high, and it can be difficult to comprehend all the things that are happening. Patients are often overwhelmed by the events that brought them to you. A warm, reassuring introduction to the unit is critical. Your role is to allay patients' fears and welcome them.

**Quick Highlight:** It's important to realize that when patients and family members are under stress, some of what you say will have to be repeated. The repetition will help to ensure that instructions and guidelines are understood.

After the introduction, focus on three additional and critical areas:

- Orientation to the room: call bell, bed operation, location of bathroom, assistive devices, etc.

- Routines: visiting hours, cafeteria operation, family services, etc.

- What's next: doctor's orders, tests, activity level, diet, etc.

Here is an example of a script to use after introduction:

"This is room 4216. Since you are next to the door, you are bed A. The phone number is 123-4567. By dialing this number, your family and friends will be connected directly to you. Our visiting hours and other information are detailed in this booklet, which I'll leave with you. Let me take a moment and explain how your bed operates and how the call bell works. During the next several hours, we will be completing the tests ordered by your physician. These tests will aid him in determining why you fainted. Let me tell you a little bit about each of them."

**Quick Highlight:** Taking time to explain the tests the patient will undergo allays anxiety and fear of the unknown. Allowing the patient to ask questions and voice his or her concerns is reassuring. By listening to the patient and family members, you build their confidence in your ability to provide needed care.

When you have completed the admission process and are preparing to leave the room, let the patient and family know:

- When you will return

- How to reach you

- That you are available to answer any questions or concerns

Here is an example of a script for when you leave Mrs. St. John:

"Mrs. St. John, do you or your family have any questions for me? I will be back to check on you in one hour. If you need me before then, just press your call bell. Is there anything else I can do for you or any other questions I can answer before I leave?"

**Quick Highlight:** Utilizing scripts during the admission process ensures that vital information will not be overlooked. For the caregiver, scripting also helps to streamline the process. Much-needed data are gathered efficiently, and consistent communication is provided to patients, family members, and other healthcare professionals.

## Summing up the admission process

Consider how you or your loved one would feel if you were unexpectedly admitted to the hospital. What information would you need, and how could the nurse help reduce your fears?

Always remember that although the verbal message is important, the non-verbal message may speak louder. Use of eye contact, tone of voice, touch, and body language are extremely important. Though we may often feel rushed and harried, every patient deserves our time and attention.

**Quick Highlight:** By consistently using scripting to welcome your patients, you can put their fears at ease, provide information for the family, start patients' experiences positively, and rarely forget important points.

Mustard, in *JONA's Healthcare Law, Ethics, and Regulation,* suggested a model for patient data collection that could be used from the first day of hospitalization to the day before discharge. His model suggests a simple and accurate way for analyzing and improving patient satisfaction by asking the patient questions about expectations while he or she is still in the hospital, rather than waiting for a postdischarge survey.

"The purpose is to identify care problems so that intervention can prevent harm and dissatisfaction. The personal interview by the nurse at the bedside during the first 24 hours after admission ... allows the hospital to know the patient's stated reasons and expectations of hospitalization" (Mustard 2003).

Mustard's model, Voice of the Patient© (see Figure 4) provides scripting for the nurse that assists in identifying patient expectations and concerns while the nurse is in a position to address them.

| Figure 4 | **Voice of the Patient**© |
|---|---|

**(PLEASE PRINT)**

**Patient name** _____

**Patient ID #** _____    **Admission date** _____

### FIRST DAY OF HOSPITALIZATION

1. What is most bothersome or troubling to you?
(One-sentence quotation)

"                                                                                          "

2. What hopes and desires do you have for this stay?
(One-sentence quotation)

"                                                                                          "

_____    _____    _____    _____
Nurse signature              Date          Attending physician signature    Date

### DAY BEFORE DISCHARGE

3a. Do you feel your hopes and desires were met for this stay?    __ Yes  __ No
3b. Would you return?                                             __ Yes  __ No

4. What hospital improvements would be most gratifying to you? (one-sentence quotation for each applicable category)
a. Convenience:        "                                                              "
b. Communication:      "                                                              "
c. Quality of care:    "                                                              "
d. Personal caring:    "                                                              "
e. Facility/equipment: "                                                              "

General comment:       "                                                              "
(experience)

_____    _____    _____    _____
Nurse signature              Date          Attending physician signature    Date

*Source: Mustard, L. (2003). Improving patient satisfaction through the consistent use of scripting by the nursing staff. JONA Healthcare, Law, & Ethics. 5(3). Used with permission.*

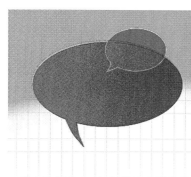

CHAPTER 3

# Daily Interactions with Patients

## Learning Objectives

After reading this chapter, you will be able to:

- Identify a tool to use in helping assess a patient's pain

- Recognize the most effective time to give patients information about discharge

- List two actions that will make you more receptive to a patient when hearing a complaint

As nurses, interacting with patients, families, and physicians is second nature. From the moment we greet our patients at the start of the shift to the time we prepare them for surgery, ready them for medical tests, discharge them, or hand them off to the next shift, we are evaluating their needs and interacting with them. Reflecting on the process makes you consciously aware of how many of those daily interactions were scripted for you in your nursing education.

Think about the simple task of introducing yourself. When you start your shift and enter a patient's room, it goes something like this: "Mr. Jones, I am Annabelle Case and I will be your nurse today." Daily, you repeat this from room to room as you make your rounds.

Quick-E! Pro: Scripting

© 2009 HCPro, Inc.

**15**

> **Quick Highlight:** Adopting scripting into your routine interactions with patients, physicians, and coworkers ensures the consistent delivery of important information.

## Managing the multitude of daily encounters

The following scenario paints a picture of a typical medical-surgical unit and some of the interactions that can take place on any given day.

It is 6:45 a.m., and you are the nurse receiving report on six patients from the offgoing nurse, Susan, on a med-surg unit. Susan reports that three of your patients are postoperative and that the other three will be going to surgery today during your shift. You review the charts of the three patients that are going to surgery and note that all the required paperwork is complete and signed.

Here's a rundown on the three postoperative patients:

■ Mrs. Talbot, a 43-year-old white female, is in room 4214 and had surgery yesterday for a cholecystectomy. She is still in quite a bit of pain and has not been out of bed yet. She was last medicated for her pain at 6:30 a.m.

■ Mr. Jones, a 73-year-old black male, is in room 4217. He is scheduled to be discharged today after undergoing surgery for a temporary ostomy six days ago. His daughter is coming in for teaching at 1:00 p.m. with the enterostomal nurse, then he will be discharged home in his daughter's care.

■ The last patient for report is Mrs. Vandemer in room 4218. She is an 81-year-old white female who underwent removal of a benign lump in her right breast yesterday. She was to be discharged last night, but had numerous complaints, and her physician postponed her discharge until today.

Let's begin with our first patient, Mrs. Talbot, and take a closer look at pain assessment.

## Discussing pain assessment

Often, one of a patient's worst fears, which can lead to great anxiety, is that he or she will be left to suffer in pain or become addicted to drugs. Communicating openly with your patient about pain control and discussing acceptable levels of pain can help reduce that anxiety. Demonstrating the use of the pain scale will help the patient in establishing his or her comfort level, as everyone tolerates pain differently. And providing information on the proper use of medications to your patient will decrease his or her fears of becoming addicted. In the following example, note how scripting is used to assess pain and establish a comfort level for Mrs. Talbot.

Mrs. Talbot was last medicated for pain at 6:30 a.m.; it is now 7:15 a.m. Upon entering her room:

- Introduce yourself. "Good morning, Mrs. Talbot. I'm Annabelle Case and I will be your nurse today."

- Acknowledge that she was recently medicated and ask about any relief since the medication was administered. "Susan told me in report that she medicated you at 6:30 a.m., and it is now 7:15 a.m. Are you feeling any relief from your pain?"

- Consider using a pain scale to evaluate her current level of pain (as shown in Figure 5). "Mrs. Talbot, on a scale of 0–10, what would you say your pain level is now?"

- Establish an acceptable pain level. "On a scale of 0–10, what do you consider a level of pain that would be acceptable at this time?"

- Reassure her that you will work with her to keep her pain at an acceptable level. "Mrs. Talbot, your doctor has written pain medication orders for you every four to six hours. Please let me know if you are starting to feel uncomfortable, and I will get you your medication."

- Comfort her before leaving the room. "Mrs. Talbot, are there any questions I can answer for you before I go? If not, I'll be back to check on you at 8:30 a.m. and assist you with getting out of bed. If you need me before that, please press your call button."

| Figure 5 | FACES pain scale |
| --- | --- |

Point to each face using the words to describe the pain intensity. Ask the patient to choose face that best describes own pain and record the appropriate number.

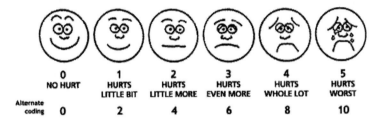

Source: From Hockenberry M.J., Wilson D., Winkelstein M.L.: Wong's Essentials of Pediatric Nursing, ed. 7, St. Louis, 2005, p. 1259. Used with permission. Copyright, Mosby

In this scenario, you conveyed a great deal of information very quickly. The patient knew who was going to be taking care of her today, that you were concerned about her pain and how she was reacting to the medication, how often she could have her medication administered if needed, when you would be back to check on her, and what was going to happen when you came back. You also reminded her to contact you with the call button if necessary. Providing your patient with information alleviates fears, addresses concerns, and conveys a message of caring.

**Quick Highlight:** Scripting your interactions brings a professional and competent presence to your relationships.

## Communicating education and discharge plans

These days, with shorter hospital stays and more complicated patient needs, it is important that we start assessing our patients for education and discharge needs on admission. Not waiting until the day of discharge provides an opportunity for the patient and family to learn each day about their care process.

In the following example, you will see Mr. Jones' postdischarge care is quite complex, and due to health and age, he will need the assistance of his daughter to ensure that he has the knowledge, skills, and supplies to make a full recovery. Had the nurse waited until the day of discharge to request teaching from the enterostomal nurse and order the needed supplies, the patient and his daughter would have been overwhelmed, and the success of his recovery could have been compromised.

**Quick Highlight:** Remember, early intervention and communication is crucial to successful discharge planning.

Let's examine how early education and planning have helped in Mr. Jones' preparation for discharge.

Mr. Jones, the patient in room 4217, is our six-day postop patient for a temporary ostomy who is awaiting discharge. Upon entering his room:

- Introduce yourself. "Good morning, Mr. Jones. I'm Annabelle Case and I will be your nurse today."

- Assess his knowledge and readiness for discharge. "Mr. Jones, you're going home today, is that correct? Who will be helping you at home with your care?"

- Acknowledge any fears or anxiety he may have about his discharge. "It is exciting to be going home. Do you have any concerns about your continued care or safety at home? I see by the note in your chart that the enterostomal nurse has been working with you in learning to care for your ostomy. Do you have any questions that I can help you with? Has your daughter picked up the supplies your doctor ordered for you?"

Because Mr. Jones was able to answer these few questions, you have identified that, with help from his daughter, he is ready for discharge. He is knowledgeable about the care of his ostomy, he has the needed supplies ready at home, and his daughter is coming in today to go over any last-minute details of his care with the enterostomal nurse. (We will discuss discharge in greater detail in Chapter 7.)

> **Quick Highlight:** Consistently following a scripted set of questions that are specifically developed for your patient population will ensure that your patients are well prepared for their experience. Nurses' ability to critically think and understand their patients' conditions will determine which questions are appropriate in a given situation.

## Hearing a patient's complaints

Despite our best efforts, patients will inevitably complain. They are scared, nervous, and sometimes angry, and they are not familiar with their surroundings. It's reasonable to think anyone in this situation would be a bit on edge.

As the nurse and the primary caregiver, it is up to you to listen to your patients' complaints and resolve them as best you can. Let's say Mrs. Vandemer, our patient in room 4218, has a few complaints about the care she's been receiving. See how scripting can be used to handle the situation.

Mrs. Vandemer is our one-day postop patient who had a benign lump removed from her right breast. Upon entering her room, introduce yourself: "Mrs. Vandemer, I'm Annabelle Case, the nurse in charge for 4 East. I understand you wanted to see me. Can you tell me about your concerns?"

**Quick Highlight:** When listening to a patient complaint, sit down if a seat is available. This lets the patient know you have time and are there to listen. The complaint may be invalid or seem trivial to you, but it is important to the patient. Remember, nonverbal actions speak volumes.

Identifying yourself as someone with authority provides the patient or family member the opportunity to voice a concern or complaint that he or she might not feel comfortable telling another staff member. Regardless of whether you are able to resolve the issue, the patient or family member has been given an opportunity to express his or her concerns. Never trivialize this interaction. Depending on the complaint, it would be appropriate to say one of the following:

- "Mrs. Vandemer, I appreciate you bringing this to my attention and I will let the department manager know of your concern."

- "Mrs. Vandemer, I'm so glad you made me aware of this. I will take steps right now to ensure that it is corrected."

- "Mrs. Vandemer, thank you for bringing this to my attention. I will investigate this further and let you know what I find."

And, as always, see whether there is anything else you can do for the patient at this point in time: "Is there anything else I can assist you with before I go?"

## Time for a timeout

Let's not forget about our patients heading to the operating room today. In an article entitled "Scripting for Success," featured in the May 2006 *AORN Journal,* author Christine Bloomfield writes that the operating room is an area that responds well to the use of scripting. The article focuses on the universal timeout prior to a surgical procedure and the scripted timeouts that reduce the likelihood of omitting any of the required elements prior to the procedure.

The Glenbrook Hospital, where Bloomfield is director of perioperative services, has adopted a timeout script (see Figure 6 on the next page) that is utilized in the operating room by all RNs in the three-hospital system.

The script takes the circulating nurse through six required elements of the timeout and ensures that all members of the surgical staff are fully engaged in the process. By using a consistent script, the process lends itself to increased patient safety and decreased risk management issues.

**Figure 6**                                                **Timeout script***

**Circulating nurse:** "This is (patient's name).""**

**Surgical team members:** "That is correct."

**Circulating nurse:** "We are doing a (left/right) (procedure) in the (position). Dr (surgeon's name), is that correct?"

**Surgeon:** "Yes."

**Circulating nurse:** "(List equipment) needed for this procedure is/are in the room. No implants are needed." Or "Implants needed for this procedure are (list implants)."

*The time out must reference six elements (i.e., patient, site and/or side, procedure, position, equipment, implants). All members of the surgical team (ie, circulating nurse, surgeon, anesthesia care provider, scrub person, all assistants) must actively participate in the time out.

**The circulating nurse reads the patient's name from the signed surgical consent form while the anesthesia care provider confirms the name with that on the patient's identity band.

*Source: Bloomfield, C. (2006). "Scripting for Success." AORN Journal May 83(5): 1127-8. Used with permission.*

As we continue through this guide, you will see other examples of how scripting can be adapted into your everyday practice.

# CHAPTER 4

# Communicating Confidently with Physicians

## Learning Objectives

After reading this chapter, you will be able to:

- List three items to have ready before calling a physician regarding a patient

- Identify two important items you should communicate to a peer in a shift report

It's a familiar scene that plays out every night across the country. Picture this:

> It is 1 o'clock in the morning. The phone rings, and a sleepy physician mumbles, "Hello?"
>
> "Dr. Bishop, this is Kelly at St. Hope's. I'm calling about your patient, Mr. Moses. He's very restless and complaining of pain that we have not been able to relieve with the medication he has ordered."
>
> "What are his vital signs?"
>
> "Ah, let me see. Oh, the assistant hasn't finished taking them yet."
>
> "When did he have his medication last?"
>
> "Let's see, it was before I got here, so I guess about 2 hours or so?"

Is it any wonder docs get frustrated? One of the biggest physician dissatisfiers is nurses calling with incomplete information. It sounds like it should be easy to fix, but it's a problem that has been around for a very long time.

**Quick Highlight:** When we're busy, stressed, or short-staffed, it's easy to forget or overlook a critical piece of information.

Scripting the nurse-physician interaction is a solution that has met with much success. Staff members and physicians have much more productive interactions when each party understands the situation fully.

## Ensure success with SBAR

You may recall we mentioned the SBAR (situation, background, assessment, and recommendation) model in Chapter 1. As we discussed, the tool is especially useful when communicating with physicians.

The Arizona Hospital and Healthcare Association went a step further and developed a "SBAR Communication Standardization in Arizona" implementation toolkit for the hospitals in the state. One piece of the toolkit, the SBAR report to the physician, is particularly helpful. (See Figure 7.) Every time a call needs to be made to a physician, this sheet is used to document the information that should be communicated. The point is that if you take just one minute to gather your thoughts along with the pertinent data, you are more likely to resolve your patient's problem.

**Figure 7** **SBAR report to physician**

**S** | **Situation**
I am calling about (patient name and location).
The problem I am calling about is _____
(I am afraid the patient is going to arrest)
**I have just assessed the patient personally.**

**Vital signs are:** BP _____ Pulse _____ Resp _____ Temp _____
I am concerned about the patient's:
__ Blood pressure because it is less          __ Color because _____
    than his acceptable systolic          __ Temperature because _____
__ Pulse because _____
__ Respiration because _____

**B** | **Background**
**The patient's mental status is:**
__ Alert and oriented to person,          __ Lethargic but able to respond and maintain
    place, and time              an airway
__ Confused          __ Stuporous and not acting or
__ Agitated or combative              talking appropriately
__ Comatose, eyes closed; not responding to stimulation

**The skin is:**
__ Warm and dry          __ Pale          __ Mottled          __ Diaphoretic
Extremities are cold or warm

**The patient is/is not on oxygen.**
O2 _____ Liters per _____ Oximeter _____
The oximeter does not detect a good pulse and is giving erratic readings.

**A** | **Assessment**
This is what I think the problem is: _____
This problem seems to be respiratory ___ cardiac ___ infection ___ neuro ___
__ I am not sure what the problem is, but the patient is deteriorating.
__ The patient seems to be unstable and may get worse; we need to do something.

**R** | **Recommendation**
**I suggest that you:**
__ Transfer to the PICU          __ Come to see the patient at this time
__ Ask for a consultant to see the patient now
**Are any tests needed:**
Do you need any tests, such as CXR, ABG, EKG, CBC, or BMP?
Others?
**If a change in treatment is ordered, then ask:**
How often do you want vital signs?
How long do you expect this problem will last?
If the patient does not get better, when would you want us to call again?

*Source: Arizona Hospital and Healthcare Association SBAR Toolkit. Used with permission.*

Although the idea isn't new, SBAR continues to catch on and improve patient care in various parts of the country. In a Robert Wood Johnson Foundation article on improving nurse-physician communication, Barbara Callahan, director of nursing education and research at North Shore–Long Island Jewish Hospital in New York, said, "Our nurses were already articulate and well informed, but SBAR has empowered them to better assess patient situations. Responses to escalating situations are now quicker, and emergency situations are dealt with faster" (Robert Wood Johnson Foundation 2009).

## Try communication cards

Some organizations use laminated cards in the nurses' station as a reminder of what information should be handy before nurses make the call. Many organizations use reminder cards similar to the one below. Note that not only has the physician conversation been scripted, but on the reverse side, the interaction between staff members when giving report has also been guided.

The front of the card, which focuses on what to do before and during a call with the physician, includes:

| | |
|---|---|
| • Getting the chart | • Identifying the patient and diagnosis |
| • Knowing whether the physician is attending, consulting, or covering | • Communicating the reason for the call |
| • Asking whether anyone else needs the physician | • Having the test results and vital signs available |
| • Confirming the correct phone number for the physician | • Summarizing what you think is going on |
| • Identifying yourself | • Saying, "I would like to suggest …" |

The back, which focuses on reports to other nurses, stresses that you should include the following:

- Patient name, age, and room number

- Attending physician and consultants

- Diagnosis and admission date with pertinent medical history

- Recent lab values, x-rays, and tests

- Postadmission critical events, interventions, and patient responses

- Current vital signs, hemodynamics—shift trends and monitor pattern

- Physical assessment, including current respiratory support

- Current support meds

- Review of lines, tubes, drains, etc.; I&O status; and daily weights

- Diet and tolerance

- Activity level

- Planned or pending labs, x-rays, tests, or procedures

- Outstanding medical orders

- Family or significant other's concerns and level of communication

- Medical and nursing goals

- Revision of care plan

Now, let's return to our initial phone call and see how it might have gone differently had Kelly been fully prepared.

It is 1 o'clock in the morning. The phone rings, and a sleepy physician mumbles, "Hello?"

"Dr. Bishop, this is Kelly at St. Hope's. I'm sorry to bother you, but I'm concerned about Mr. Moses. He's very restless and complaining of pain that we have not been able to relieve with the medication he has ordered. His order is for Demerol 50 mg IM every 4 hours PRN. His last dose was 2 hours ago. His blood pressure is 190/100; his respirations and pulse are elevated. His lungs are clear, and he is not diaphoretic. His temperature is normal, and there is no unusual drainage from his incision. Mr. Moses is a large man— his weight this morning prior to surgery was 280 pounds. I'd like to get an order to give him an additional dose of his pain medication ahead of schedule, and we'll monitor him closely for any changes in vital signs."

"Kelly, thanks for the call. I agree with your thorough assessment and think you're absolutely right. Let's go ahead and give him another 50 mg of Demerol IM now. Let's also change his pain medication order to Demerol 75 mg IM every 4 hours PRN. Do you need anything else?"

"No, I'm confident this will improve his comfort level. We'll monitor his vital signs and see you in the morning."

"Great. See you about 7."

This time, there was more information, which provided less frustration for the physician. Using a scripted process ensures that the nurse is ready with the data the physician will need to make an informed decision and increases the likelihood that the communication will be successful.

## Facing face-to-face interactions

This scripted process does not apply to only phone conversations. When the physician appears on your unit, he or she expects that you will be as well informed in person as you were on the phone. Using the same scripted format to organize your patient data will give you a built-in, ready-made report for the physician no matter when he or she arrives.

**Quick Highlight:** What often gets in the way of nurse-physician communi-cation has more to do with style than information. Physicians are trained to be problem solvers. They want their information delivered in short, to-the-point facts. Nursing education leans toward creating professionals who are narrative and detailed.

Let's look to the following scenario as an example:

Dr. Pitt has arrived on the unit to make rounds. "Where's Gloria? I'm in a hurry and I've got to see my patients and get to the OR."

"She's in Mrs. Anderson's room. I'll let her know you're here," the unit clerk responds.

Two to three minutes pass. It is clear that Dr. Pitt is not a patient person.

Gloria rounds the corner to the nurses' station, and Dr. Pitt pounces. "Let's go. I've got three cases today and I need to get down to the OR [without taking a breath]. Tell me what's going on with Anderson, Clive, and Webster."

**Does panic set in, or have you methodically prepared for this moment all morning?**

Calmly, Gloria pulls the needed charts and, drawing from her scripted dialog, begins to give Dr. Pitt the information he needs. She knows that he makes rounds every day and that he's interested in the following changes since yesterday's rounds:

- Any lab values that have recently come back (especially outliers)

- Test results that have recently come back

- The general condition of his patients (comfort, pain relief, wound status, etc.)

- Whether the patients are meeting their recovery goals in preparation for discharge

- Whether the patients need anything to begin discharge preparation

"Gloria, thanks again," says Dr. Pitt. "You're always ready for me. I'll be in the OR if you need me."

Building that relationship didn't happen overnight. Trust and respect are built over time.

**Quick Highlight:** The first time you meet another caregiver, introduce yourself and let him or her know you're interested in being as supportive as possible. Each individual on your care team can benefit from a scripted interaction that speaks to his or her need for information.

**Quick Highlight:** Improving communication between physicians and nurses has many benefits. Not only is patient care and satisfaction positively affected, but there is also increased trust and respect between physicians and nurses. Subsequently, you will create a positive communication model, and collaborative practice is enhanced.

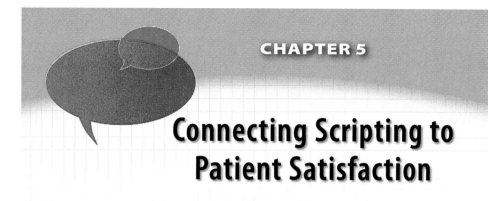

# CHAPTER 5

# Connecting Scripting to Patient Satisfaction

## Learning Objectives

After reading this chapter, you will be able to:

- Discuss the "5 on the Board" program that improved patient satisfaction scores at CHRISTUS Hospital–St. Mary's in Port Arthur, TX

- Identify questions gathered by mystery shoppers that helped keep patient satisfaction scores high at CHRISTUS Hospital–St. Mary's

- List two additional ways to improve patient satisfaction scores

- Identify an appropriate comment to begin the process of delivering bad news to a patient

In the past few chapters, we have discussed the use of scripting in the everyday practice of bedside nursing and in other hospital areas, such as environmental services and the operating room. Now we'll take a closer look at how scripting is connected to patient satisfaction.

# Case study: Turning the patient satisfaction tide in Texas

In 2005, CHRISTUS Hospital–St. Mary's in Port Arthur, TX, was faced
with patient satisfaction scores at an all-time low of 33% (*www.strategiesfor-
nursemanagers.com*). This deeply concerned the hospital's administration.
Challenged with turning the scores around, the nursing directors and managers came to the table to find ways to improve patient satisfaction. They were
on a limited budget and were faced with a tight time frame. One of the key
drivers was making directors and managers the key stakeholders. It was
their job to ensure that their units implemented the initiatives and held staff
members accountable for the change process.

Scripting was the answer.

The nursing managers started making daily rounds on all of the patients on
their units. By asking scripted questions of their patients, the nurse managers
learned what was working and what wasn't. When entering patients' rooms,
nurse managers identified themselves as managers and gave their names. They
also provided business cards so the patient would be able to get in touch if they
had questions or concerns. During their conversation, managers would ask
patients to rate their quality of care on a scale of 1–5, with 5 being very good.
As part of the initiative St. Mary's named "5 on the Board," the score was then
placed on the patients' white boards and was visible to all staff members. If
patients gave scores lower than 5, managers would ask them, "What can I do to
improve that score?" The managers, along with their staff members, would
then take steps to meet those requests.

For example, a patient had been served green beans at lunch for two days, even
though he disliked them. In response to his complaint, the nurse manager

called dietary to make the staff aware of the patient's request, and he didn't get green beans again during his stay. Making the phone call to dietary right from the room made an impression on the patient by showing that his needs were important, even if the issue was as small as not liking his vegetables.

The implementation of this program is a nice example of the usefulness of scripting. Additionally, it is important to note the program's overall, long-term success. After one year, the hospital's patient satisfaction scores rose to the 90% range. St. Mary's kept the momentum going through the use of mystery shoppers.

The mystery shoppers would visit patients where issues had been reported and ask them four scripted questions:

1. "I see you have a 5 on your board. Who did that?"

2. "Have you met your manager today?"

3. "Has your manager made rounds every day?"

4. "Do you know what that 5 on your board means?"

The information gathered by the mystery shoppers was then shared with the guest relations manager for follow-up.

St. Mary's program was so successful that it received the health system's Touchstone Award for its efforts and became a model of excellence for the entire healthcare organization.

# Quick ways to improve patient satisfaction scores

Looking for some other simple, effective ways to help improve patient satisfaction scores at your organization?

Here are a few popular suggestions from an online nursing social network:

- **Hourly rounding.** It may seem difficult, but it's actually easy. Nurses can do even hours, and aides can do the odd. Leave a note or write on the white board if patients are asleep.

- **Say good-bye.** When you're leaving for the day/night, stop to say good-bye and let patients know who will be assuming their care.

- **Answer the call light in 30 seconds or less.** Whoever is closest to the desk should answer the light, find out what is needed, and carry out the request. The key is to follow through.

**Quick Highlight:** There are many ways to meet patients' needs and improve their satisfaction that cost nothing to implement.

Press Ganey's 2008 national survey of hospital executives (*www.hfma.org*) found that organizations focused on patient satisfaction for the following major reasons:

- Improving the quality of care

- Measuring loyalty

- Increasing market share

The hospitals with the healthiest bottom line also had high levels of patient satisfaction—hence the push to keep those scores high.

Nurses have always played a key role in the patients' perception of quality of care. Promoting a culture of safety by using scripting in handoffs (as discussed in Chapter 4) or during shift transitions provides patients with a high level of patient satisfaction.

## A guideline for delivering bad news

In nursing school, you probably didn't learn the "how-tos" of delivering bad news to patients and families. Often, we are left to learn by seeing others do it. Over time, we are exposed to those who do it well and those who do not. Scripting can help guide your ability to prepare for these difficult times.

The following is a quick, four-step guide:

1.   Prepare yourself. Think about whom you will be speaking with, what you want to say, and whether you have all the information necessary for the conversation.

2.   When you're ready to deliver the news, be as straightforward as possible. Provide for privacy (e.g., the patient's room or a waiting room). HIPAA guidelines require privacy and confidentiality, but guidelines aside, this is a vulnerable time for the patient and family, and their dignity should be respected. The people for whom we provide care are from various cultures and walks of life; we can never predict how each person will respond to bad news.

3.   Choose the right words to say. For example, open the conversation with "I'm sorry to have to tell you this ..." or, "I wish I had better news to share with you ..."

4.  Once you have explained the news, you can express your own sadness while reassuring the patient or family that you and the staff are here to help them through this. For example, offer consolation to a grieving family by saying, "I was with him when he died; he was not alone." This comforts the family and often helps relieve any guilt felt by not being present.

**Quick Highlight:** "Breaking bad news is an on-the-job skill learned only in the doing, in the holding of patients' hands and in simple comforting acts that suddenly erase the distance between patient/family and caregiver: the hug that keeps someone on their feet; the way we sometimes let patients/families see tears in our own eyes" (Davis 2008).

**Quick Highlight:** Giving bad news is never a pleasant task, but it's one in which the delivery is important and long remembered.

## Providing direction in the hospital

Hospital campuses are often very spread out, sometimes covering multiple city blocks, and often, we encounter a patient or family member in the hall who has lost his or her way. Assisting those folks who find themselves lost and confused can promote a culture of caring in your institution.

Again, a few scripted phrases make this an easy customer service win. Staff members who are helpful, courteous, and knowledgeable are perceived as caring.

Consider the following tips:

- Approach a lost patient or family member by saying, "Excuse me, do you need assistance in finding your way?"

- Rather than simply giving directions, take the person to where he or she needs to go, if possible. Escorting the patient or family member will leave him or her with a strong positive impression.

- If you don't know how to get the person to his or her destination, you might say something such as, "I am not familiar with where that is located. Let's walk over to that office and we'll find the way."

Patients, families, and visitors may not say so, but they do notice when people make the extra effort—and they will tell others. Taking the extra step with something as simple as giving directions to someone who is lost aids in building recognition and loyalty to your organization.

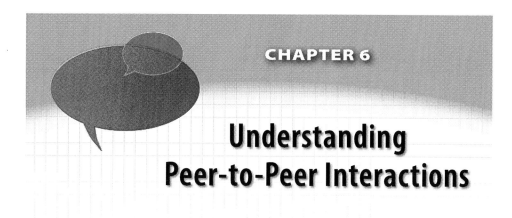

# CHAPTER 6

# Understanding Peer-to-Peer Interactions

## Learning Objectives

After reading this chapter, you will be able to:

- Identify three of the most frequently reported negative behaviors by new nurses

- List two appropriate statements to make when you feel you are being ignored

- Choose an appropriate statement to make when thanking support personnel members for their help

Effective communication between peers is complex. Emotions, thoughts, and reactions to what is seen and heard are intertwined with spoken words and personal beliefs. Often, in the emotion of the moment, words are spoken that are harsh or hurtful. When this happens, barriers begin to form that can result in hostile work environments.

**Quick Highlight:** Even if negative words are not spoken, tone of voice and/or body language can communicate negativity.

# Using scripting in negative situations

Horizontal violence is a term used in today's literature to describe the overt and covert behaviors nurses sometimes use toward their peers and coworkers. Using a few good phrases in situations in which you are the recipient of or witness to horizontal violence can give you ammunition to disarm offenders professionally and hold them accountable for their actions. Additionally, scripting can help you avoid using negativity to address a problem with a peer.

Consider the following scenario:

Berta is an experienced med-surg nurse and has worked the day shift for the past 12 years. Nancy has three years of experience and recently transferred from nights to the day shift on the same unit. She asks Berta for help getting an IV restarted on one of her patients who is a difficult "stick." Nancy walks into the room while Berta is starting the IV. She notices that Berta is not wearing any gloves. Nancy hesitates, wondering how to approach Berta about her unsafe practice.

**What would you say?**

As a professional, Nancy has an obligation to call attention to Berta's unsafe practice, but doing so in this example may cause conflict. Nancy has less tenure on the unit and is still trying to fit in on the day shift. Ideally, though, tenure and years of experience should not play into this conversation because Berta's actions are wrong and unsafe. Universal precautions are to be practiced each and every time there is a reasonable chance to come into contact with blood or body fluids. It would border on unethical behavior to ignore this breach of protocol. Using a scripted phrase or approach can make it easier to begin the conversation.

> **Quick Highlight:** Anytime you need to confront a peer—or anyone, for that matter—about a problem you have with him or her, the best practice is to pull the person aside as soon as possible after the event and hold the conversation in private.

Reimagining this scenario, if Nancy enters the room while Berta is preparing to initiate the IV and notices Berta is not wearing gloves, one option is to simply hand Berta a pair of gloves and say in a light tone, "Here you go, Berta. Don't forget these." If Nancy enters the room after Berta has initiated the IV, she might say, "Berta, I noticed you didn't wear any gloves when you started Mr. Hagg's IV. Can you tell me why?" or, "Berta, I am worried about your safety. I noticed you weren't wearing any gloves when you started Mr. Hagg's IV."

Expressing your concern for maintaining your peer's safety or the safety of the patient can divert the negative emotion of being caught performing in an unsafe way and focus on the positive emotion of protecting or helping to preserve the safety of the situation.

## Handling negative reactions to confrontation

Let's imagine the previous scenario playing out negatively. Berta may not be receptive to suggestions or invitations to practice safely. What if she responds to Nancy unprofessionally, making the situation more difficult? For example, Berta might say, "I know what I'm doing," or, "If you don't like the way I start your IVs, then you can start them yourself."

Frequently, situations such as these escalate into conflicts that, if left unresolved, cause staff members to become divided. Subsequently, morale begins to suffer. When a staff member feels his or her knowledge base is being challenged, he or she may not say anything at the time, but the staff member's body language and conversations with other peers may have just as much of a negative effect on group cohesiveness as confrontation.

According to findings from a study by Stevenson, Randle, and Grayling (2006), the most frequently reported negative behaviors experienced by new nurses are:

- Being ignored or excluded

- Being criticized

- Resentment

- Humiliation

- Perceiving that their efforts are not valued

- Being teased

Figure 8 lists some scripted phrases for these negative behaviors and difficult conversations.

**Figure 8** **Scripts for difficult conversations**

| Situation | Script |
|---|---|
| Practice variation/ being criticized | "Can you explain to me why you did [procedure] that way and not by protocol?" |
| | "Let me show you the method that the protocol/policy describes. I'm sure you'll see why it's important to do it this way." |
| | "Do you want to show/tell me how you would have done it/how you would have handled the situation?" |
| Being ignored | "I understand you're busy. What can I do to help?" |
| | "Excuse me, I'd like to help/participate." |
| | "I can come back in 10 minutes if that works better for you." |
| Feelings of resentment/ personal conflicts | "I'm trying to do my best, but I need to …" |
| | "Please help me understand why you feel this way." |
| | "Can we discuss this in the breakroom? I would like to understand what I did to upset you." |
| | "We all need to work together. Can we find a compromise/common ground so we can move forward?" |
| Being teased or humiliated | "I don't understand why you did [action]. Can you explain to me?" |
| | "Please help me understand why …" |
| | "I'm sorry you feel/think/believe that. What can I do to change your perception?" |
| | "I heard what you said to [person A] about [person B]. I think we should talk and figure things out. We all need to work together." |
| | "That hurt my feelings. Can we sit down and talk about this? We need to work this out." |

Negative or hostile work environments are not only difficult to work in and cause low morale, but they are also dangerous for patients. When this kind of environment is present, patient satisfaction declines, and the rate of errors rises (Ramos 2006).

 **Quick Highlight:** Nurses must feel empowered to speak up and deal with any peer-to-peer negativity before it escalates and affects patient safety or satisfaction.

Whenever you decide it is appropriate to use a script, you must be sure you:

- Respect the other person's right to have a different point of view.

- Use "I" statements instead of "you" statements. This removes the feeling of being attacked and does not put the other person on the defense.

- Speak clearly and sincerely to allow the other person to feel comfortable responding.

It's important to understand that there may be some situations that simply are not resolvable at the peer level. When this is the case, it is appropriate to engage the chain of command at your workplace. Engaging the chain of command usually entails notifying your immediate supervisor that an unresolvable problem exists between yourself and a peer or that a peer is taking an action that carries the possibility of causing harm to a patient or coworker. Examples of such events include:

- Not identifying a patient before administering a medication

- Not wearing the proper protective devices when performing a procedure

It may seem like you are being a tattletale, but if you consider what the consequences might be if left uncorrected, notifying your supervisor is the right thing to do.

> **Quick Highlight:** If you are observing something that could result in harm to a patient or coworker, don't hesitate to speak up!

## The power of reinforcing positive actions

Have you ever felt that you've done a great job and no one noticed? Have you ever seen someone else do something exceptional, but were too timid to say anything? Unfortunately, people are usually quick to jump at a chance to find fault or something that wasn't done correctly, but they're not so quick to say "great job." What about the article you just read in a professional journal that you believe has value for your peers, or that conference you attended where you picked up some good information about a problem your unit has been experiencing? These are the positive moments in nursing that are often missed because we are too busy finding fault.

Let's look back to Berta and Nancy and play out their scenario a bit differently. Recall that Berta has 12 years of experience on med-surg; Nancy is new to the day shift but has three years of med-surg experience on nights. Nancy has asked Berta for help getting a difficult IV restarted on one of her patients. Berta is able to restart the IV without much difficulty, but seems to be annoyed with Nancy. What would you say?

Let's consider some ways Nancy might approach Berta. She could say any of the following:

- "Thank you, Berta, for taking the time to help me. Is there anything I can help you with?"

- "Berta, you must show me how you are able to handle these difficult patients!"

- "Berta, thank you for getting that IV started! The patient really needed her fluids. I know my patient thanks you, too."

However, as powerful as it can be, saying "thank you" in excess (if there is such a thing) can diminish the value and perceived sincerity of the words. Reinforcing your words with a short note or a token of gratitude, such as a favorite candy bar in your peer's locker or an offer to buy a soda or snack, is a good way to demonstrate the sincerity of your words.

When a peer is recognized by another peer for doing something positive, the gesture is priceless. It can erase many negatives that may have occurred during a shift. Often, we become so engaged in our own assignments and challenges that we do not think about the simple value of saying "thanks" or "good job." Figure 9 is a collection of phrases that are adaptable to times or situations in which positive peer reinforcement is appropriate.

| Figure 9 | Scripts for positive reinforcement |

| Situation | Script |
|---|---|
| Handling a difficult patient or family member | "I watched how you dealt with [patient/family member/etc.] today. You were very effective." |
| Emotional/difficult situation | "It must have been hard for you to deal with [situation]. You did well." |
| Presentation to group | "Your [poster/presentation/etc.] was very informative. I got a lot out of it." |
| Physician concerns | "Dr. [name] can be difficult at times. You handled the situation [well/professionally]." |

## Treat support personnel with respect

Although this subcategory is listed separately, there should be little difference between how the professional nurse interacts with the ancillary and support staff and how he or she treats peers.

**Quick Highlight:** The basic principle of effective communication is respect. If you are respectful of people and the jobs they do, your communication scripts should not deviate much from the examples we have demonstrated earlier in this chapter. The negative situations described are not unique to nurses. Nursing techs, nurse aides, radiology techs, and dietary aides—just to name a few—all have conflicts with each other and with nurses. As a nurse, you may find yourself playing mediator when conflict exists between two support personnel, but when the negative situation occurs between yourself and an ancillary or support staff member, you must take the high road, be professional, and lead the dialog using effective communication.

When using a suggested script with ancillary or support staff, be careful not to sound condescending. Avoid using medical jargon or technical terminology unless you are sure the recipient has a sound knowledge of the terminology. If English is not their primary language, speak clearly and slowly to allow them the time to process the words.

After finishing a thought or sentence, you may want them to repeat back to you what it is they understood: "Before I leave, I want to be sure you understand. Can you tell me in your own words what I just told you?"

Use the same courtesy and professional respect you would when speaking with a peer, regardless of the position the support staff or ancillary staff holds. You may refer back to Figures 8 and 9 for scripting examples. Just remember to edit some of the terminology to simpler terms as appropriate.

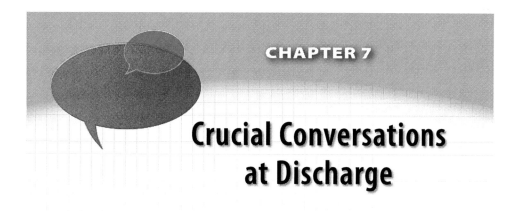

# Crucial Conversations at Discharge

## Learning Objectives

After reading this chapter, you will be able to:

- Identify how scripting can help with the HCAHPS hospital survey

- Explain how to use the mnemonic device "HEART" when discharging a patient

Today's hospital stays are whirlwind experiences for many patients. It can seem that as soon as they are admitted, they are discharged. In between these two moments, nurses must ensure that patients receive discharge instruction that covers not only their medical condition, but also medications, diet changes, dressing or wound care (if applicable), and plans for follow-up care. Nurses should use every appropriate moment to educate their patients.

**Quick Highlight:** Becoming familiar and comfortable with scripting can facilitate the discharge process.

# Providing effective patient education

Whenever possible, plan for uninterrupted teaching time, but always look for appropriate moments that might present themselves during routine care. They can be excellent for initial instruction.

For example, let's say you are entering the room to hang a piggyback medication. The patient asks, "What's that for?" This is a perfect time for you to respond by answering the question and add, "You will need to continue taking this medication in tablet form when you go home. Why don't I finish this, get some written materials for you, and return after lunch so we can go over what you need to know in more detail?"

The following are some additional principles for excellent discharge teaching:

- Sit down and maintain good eye contact with the patient.

- Acknowledge that the patient may already know about his or her condition or medication. Validate that what the patient knows is correct.

- Do not appear rushed. Try to plan for a time when you will not be interrupted.

- Take advantage of the "teachable moment" whenever you can.

- Acknowledge when the patient seems to have had enough information for one episode and ask when he or she might want to go over the information again. Be sure to document the patient's response and pass it along to the next caregiver.

Let's look at a scenario where some scripted phrases can help to initiate your discharge teaching. Mrs. Canterberry is a 78-year-old retired school teacher who was admitted yesterday with congestive heart failure. She is responding well to the therapies ordered, and her physician plans on discharging her tomorrow. She will need to continue her diuretic and a potassium supplement in addition to the antihypertensive medication she has been on for years. She will also need to monitor her weight daily and learn how to manage her sodium intake.

Start the conversation by talking about the patient's diagnosis and symptoms. This is the first thing on the patient's mind and his or her biggest worry, so you want to begin with the most important information. (In our example, we will continue to use Mrs. Canterberry. Just substitute accordingly with your own patients and conditions.)

Here are a few talking points regarding Mrs. Canterberry's diagnosis and symptoms:

- "Tell me what you know about congestive heart failure."

- "I know it is scary and overwhelming. Let me try to explain heart failure to you."

- "I know you've been diagnosed with high blood pressure for some time. Can you tell me what you already know about it?"

- "Here is some information for you to look at. I'll be back later to go over it with you and answer any questions you may have."

If time is not on your side, be sure to supply the patient with written information and review its critical elements. You may also give the patient other information, such as a Web site or the phone numbers of community resources, to refer back to once he or she is discharged and home.

The next crucial subjects to cover are medications and treatments. After patients understand their condition, they need to know their postdischarge treatment plan. They will want to know how and when they are going to feel better, or how their lives will change. For example, the following are a few talking points regarding Mrs. Canterberry's medications and treatments:

- "The doctor has prescribed Lasix to help remove the excess fluid from your body. Let me give you some important information about it."

- "Here is some written information about Lasix. I will return after lunch to go over it with you."

- "It is important for you to take this medication exactly as it is prescribed. Would it be helpful if we worked out a schedule for you to use at home?"

- "You will need to limit your salt intake."

- "I have a list of foods you should avoid or limit. Why don't you look through it and circle any that are favorites of yours? This way, we can look at ways to modify your use of them."

- "One way to know if your medications are working and your diet is right is to weigh yourself at the same time every day and write the results in a small notebook."

Many patients think that when they are discharged from the hospital, they are better and there is no need to see the doctor unless they get sick again. An important part of discharge teaching is prevention and/or maintenance of patients' conditions.

**Quick Highlight:** Staying in close contact with their physician or medical team might not be at the front of your patients' minds, but be sure to convey how important it is to their recovery.

You may not have exact information regarding the postdischarge care plan until the day of discharge. Should the patient ask before this information is known, it is appropriate to respond, "I'm not aware of your physician's exact plan for you, but I know it is important for patients diagnosed with [condition] to be closely monitored by their doctor."

For example, the following are a few talking points regarding Mrs. Canterberry's follow-up care:

- "It is important that you make a follow-up appointment with your doctor within one week."

- "Continuous medical monitoring is needed for congestive heart failure. Please be sure you make and keep your appointments with your doctor."

- "Do you have a way to get to your appointments?"

- "If you feel short of breath or have a sudden weight gain [or other appropriate symptoms], you must notify your doctor immediately."

**Quick Highlight:** Effective discharge instruction that is centered on and understandable by the patient can make the difference in his or her ability to prevent a reoccurrence of symptoms and rehospitalizations. With chronic conditions, solid discharge instruction can increase patients' quality of life by ensuring that they have the information needed to manage their lives better.

# Good scripting can lead to a good rating

The Hospital Consumer Assessment of Healthcare Providers and Systems (HCAHPS) hospital survey was launched in 2006 by Centers for Medicare & Medicaid Services and the Agency for Healthcare Research and Quality to standardize patient satisfaction surveys across the nation.

In addition, some facilities employ the services of a private customer satisfaction survey service. Whether this is Press Ganey, Gallup, or a homegrown satisfaction survey, your "last words" can have a positive effect on how patients or their families complete the survey.

The questions asked by HCAHPS are available on its Web site. The private satisfaction survey should be available to you, but you may have to ask for it. If you are aware of the questions asked on the survey, you can speak to patients using language that they will be able to recognize when taking the survey. It's almost like an open-book test.

If you know the survey asks, "How often did the nurses treat you with courtesy and respect?" then you know you must use phrases such as "I respect your right to refuse this medication, but I want to be sure you understand how important it is for you." Knowing the questions allows you, at discharge, to summarize them in a short paragraph and try to "remind" patients and/or their families of the "right" answers. Figure 10 shows a selection of HCAHPS questions and some scripts related to each.

**Figure 10**                                                    **Scripts for HCAHPS questions**

| HCAHPS Question | Suggested Script |
|---|---|
| How often did the nurse listen carefully to you? | "I hear what you are saying." |
|  | "If I heard you correctly, you want ..." |
| After you pressed the call button, how often did you get help as soon as you wanted it? | "Mr. Jones, please don't wait until your pain is severe. Call me as soon as it feels like it's reaching [level] so I can respond in time." |
| How often was the area around your room quiet at night? | "May I close your door so you will not be disturbed by any noise?" |
| Did the doctors or nurses talk with you about whether you had the help you needed when you left the hospital? | "I'm concerned about how you will manage at home. Who is available to help you?" |
|  | "I can ask the case manager to come in and talk with you about arranging to have some help when you get home if that is okay with you." |

**Quick Highlight:** Regardless of the reason you are in the patient's room (excluding emergency situations), one scripted phrase that will serve you well in most situations is simply asking the patient, "Is there anything else I can do for you?" Needless to say, when these words are spoken, they must be sincere and caring. All the scripting in the world cannot hide a poor attitude.

## Be sure to summarize—and simplify—instructions

The time of discharge is an excellent chance to review everything that has happened during the course of the hospitalization, make final attempts to reconcile loose ends or missed opportunities, and summarize the instruction that has occurred.

Returning to Mrs. Canterberry and her diagnosis of congestive heart failure, let's explore some scripting for her discharge. Any of the following statements are appropriate and effective when leaving a patient for the last time:

- "Mrs. Canterberry, can we review one last time what you need to know when you go home?"

- "I'm so pleased that you have made such a quick recovery; please take care of yourself. Remember what we talked about?"

- "Do you have those handouts I gave you about your medications and diet? Remember to refer to them if you have questions."

- "Before you leave, are there any questions you need me to answer?"

Discharge is a good time to ensure that any misconceptions or misunderstandings have been fully resolved. Some sincere, well-scripted phrases can make you look like a professional conflict mediator. A simple mnemonic to use is HEART:

- **H**ear your patient. Look at and listen to what he or she is saying.

- **E**mpathize with the concern. Say, "I can understand that this made you feel …"

- **A**pologize that the incident happened. Say, "I'm sorry you experienced [problem]."

- **R**espond. Say, "Let me see what I can do," or, "I am not sure what the answer is, but I will look into this and get back to you."

- **T**hank the patient for the opportunity to help him or her resolve the situation.

**Quick Highlight:** Taking ownership and responsibility for fixing a problem can give patients the impression that their concerns are taken seriously and their opinions count. None of us want to feel like we do not matter, despite how trivial an issue might seem.

Finally, when all the paperwork has been completed and the patient is dressed and ready to leave the facility, you must say good-bye. Often, facilities have transport personnel or a unit technician or aide push the wheelchair or escort the patient to the car.

Therefore, the bedside is the last opportunity to express your professionalism. Be sure to thank the patient and call him or her by name. Say, "Thank you, Mrs. Canterberry, for letting me care for you," or, "It was my pleasure to care for you, Mrs. Canterberry. I hope you continue to have a speedy recovery."

Additionally, if family members are present, an added statement to them is often appropriate, such as "Your mother has been a pleasure to care for. She is a special lady."

Remember, giving patients instructions about their care while in the hospital and instructions on how to maintain their health after being discharged is important not only for their health, but also their satisfaction.

**Quick Highlight:** Using scripting can help you tell patients the right things at the right times, defuse conflict, and increase patient satisfaction.

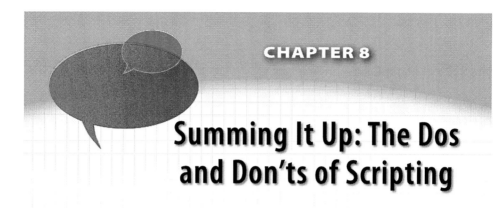

# CHAPTER 8

# Summing It Up: The Dos and Don'ts of Scripting

## Learning Objectives

After reading this chapter, you will be able to:

■ Identify when scripting should not be used

The previous chapters in this book have described scripting examples to assist you in your day-to-day communication. Remember that scripting is a tool to help create meaningful conversations with your peers, physicians, and your patients. Let's finish up by looking at some of the dos and don'ts of scripting.

## Forget about memorization

Rote memorization and recitation of scripted phrases is not what good communication is about. You likely remember having a bedtime story recited to you as a child. The desired effect of the story was for you to drift off to sleep. You may find the same thing happening to your listener if you deliver scripted phrases in a "reading out loud" tone of voice.

**Quick Highlight:** Whenever you use scripting, it must seem spontaneous and reflect what you know and believe. You do not want to sound like a robot that's programmed to say certain things when prompted by certain cues.

Let's look at two example deliveries of a script. Version A is recited; version B is spontaneous:

- **Version A.** "Mr. Jones, my name is Mary, and I need to start an IV on you. Can you please tell me your full name and date of birth so I can verify that I have the right patient?" [Mr. Jones states his full name and birth date.] "Thank you, Mr. Jones. Now may I please see your arms?"

- **Version B.** "Good morning, Mr. Jones. How are you feeling today? My name is Mary, and I will be your nurse today. The doctor wants to give you some intravenous medicine, so I need to look for a good vein and start an IV line on you. Before I start, I need to verify that I have the correct patient. Can you please tell me your full name and date of birth?" [Mr. Jones states his full name and birth date.] "Thanks! Now let's get looking for your best vein."

Both versions of this script convey the same information. Nothing incorrect or inappropriate was said in version A, but version B sounds more relaxed and caring. Imagine that you are Mr. Jones. Who would you rather have start your IV: the person who recited version A, or the person who was compassionate and communicative in version B?

**Quick Highlight:** When scripting sounds forced, patients may perceive you as stiff or rushed. They may think you are uncaring or have no concern for their situation.

Nonverbal communication is real. You might say all the right things, but your nonverbal communication—body language and tone of voice—will make either a positive or negative impression on your patient.

Research shows that up to 55% of communication is nonverbal. Experts estimate that, of that number, 38% is tone of voice. The actual words spoken comprise only 7% of communication. Thus, it is important for you to be aware that although your words (scripts) may say one thing, your voice and body may be saying something else.

Look at the behaviors in Figure 11 and identify the things you find yourself doing when speaking with patients, peers, or physicians. Use this knowledge to modify how your body speaks when you are interacting with these individuals (Navarro 2008).

Figure 11 |

| Impression | Actions |
|---|---|
| Nervousness/tension | • Fidgeting of hands or feet<br>• Avoiding eye contact (unless for a cultural reason)<br>• Jingling keys or change in pocket/hands in pockets<br>• Tugging at ears<br>• Clicking your pen |
| Confidence/enthusiasm | • Open hands, unhidden in pockets<br>• Chin upward<br>• Firm gaze/constant eye contact<br>• Sitting on edge of chair<br>• Moving closer |
| Defensiveness | • Looking down or away<br>• Hand to cheek, leaning back<br>• No eye contact<br>• Arms crossed on chest<br>• Locked (crossed) ankles<br>• Gripping a wrist |
| Contemplation/thought | • Stroking chin<br>• Pinching bridge of nose<br>• Glancing upward<br>• Open hand to cheek<br>• Taking off glasses |
| Boredom/disinterest | • Doodling<br>• Head in hand<br>• Turning body toward exit<br>• Blank stare<br>• Leaning back or away |

## Settle in with scripting

The first time your nurse leader tells you that scripting will be used at your facility, a frequent reaction is to lash out with feelings of anger or resentment. You might think, "They can't make me say anything I don't feel comfortable saying," or, "Scripting is stupid. It's just a way for 'them' to tell us how to practice." Neither of these statements is true. The feelings may be real, but the fact is that scripting can be an excellent tool to help staff members communicate the right information at the right time.

We practice in a world where there is a great deal of research being conducted. No longer is it appropriate to defend a practice by saying, "That's the way we've always done it." Several studies have shown that effective communication between the patient and the caregiver improves patient satisfaction and safety.

Using scripting as a way to promote effective communication can improve satisfaction, so put away your doubts and give it a try. Whether you are a new or seasoned nurse, it is understandable if you initially feel uncomfortable and stammer a bit in getting the phrases out smoothly. Starting with scripting can resemble learning a foreign language: the words come out slowly and purposefully, but without a smooth flow. Keep practicing the phrases, and they will become as easy and fluid as your native tongue.

**Quick Highlight:** Although it may seem corny, try writing down a scripted phrase. Work with the words—change them around and substitute them with others that have similar meanings. Then try the new script on for size. You may find that if you customize the script, you'll like it better and use it more frequently.

Any therapeutic conversation between healthcare providers (peer-to-peer, nurse-to-physician, etc.) or between providers and patients has a purpose. Whether it is informative or instructional, our days are filled with receiving and giving information. Between these moments, nurses must analyze data, be constantly alert to changes in their patients' conditions, advocate for patients' wishes and needs, and decide on appropriate nursing interventions. With so much to do and think about, wouldn't it be nice to be able to have an effortless therapeutic conversation using scripted phrases?

## Avoid scripting in the wrong environments

Throughout this book, we have outlined situations in which scripting can be used to improve nurse-patient, nurse-physician, and nurse-nurse communication. But there is one time that scripts should NOT be used: emergency situations. Emergencies require responders to react immediately.

Looking at a typical emergency scenario, we can see that there is little room for scripting.

Imagine that Helen, a nurse's aide, enters a patient's room to take routine vital signs and finds the patient cyanotic and unresponsive. She begins to yell, "Help! Help!" You and another nurse respond by running down to see what's happening. Once you arrive, do you draw upon your script and ask, "Helen, can you tell me what's happening?" or do you look at the patient and tell Helen to call a code while you and the other nurse start CPR? The answer is obvious. There may be a time for scripting after the emergency, when you are interacting with the family or debriefing with the code team. These times can be stressful, and scripts can lessen the stress, but in the moment of the actual emergency, it's best to let instinct take over.

Earlier, we discussed that being comfortable with scripting will improve how you are perceived by the listener. It's important to keep in mind that the opposite effect will occur when using a script incorrectly or in the wrong situation.

For example, imagine you are communicating with a patient who has been admitted with a substance abuse issue. The patient is agitated and having withdrawal symptoms that are not being adequately controlled by the ordered medications. In this situation, it makes little sense to rely on a script and ask, "What can I do to help you?" or say, "Please quiet down, you're disturbing the other patients."

**Quick Highlight:** Using scripted lines when the patient is excited or agitated will usually only make the situation worse.

Just like running a successful business, location plays into the success or failure of an interaction. Having the right conversation in the wrong location can have disastrous consequences. As an example, imagine that you have just witnessed a peer violate policy. The violation is severe enough that you feel you must bring this to his or her attention before a serious event happens. Without thinking, you approach your peer in the middle of the nurses' station. Stop. Look around. If the tables were turned, would you want to be in this situation, where everyone nearby can hear what is being said?

The best scripting cannot make up for choosing the wrong location or having poor timing. It's best to find a private area, such as the nurses' lounge or a conference room, to speak with a peer or coworker about a sensitive issue.

**Quick Highlight:** If the conversation is headed in a direction that might involve legal ramifications (e.g., HR issues or breaches in the standard of care), have a neutral witness present that can validate what was said.

When speaking to a patient or family member about sensitive material (including any health information), it's best to wait for another time if there are visitors in the room. If the conversation cannot wait, ask the visitors to step out for a moment.

For example, say to the patient, "Mr. Jones, I need to go over some important information with you. Is it okay if I ask your visitors to step out for a moment? It should only take five to 10 minutes." Then address the visitors: "There is a waiting area at the end of this hall if you would like to wait there, or the cafeteria makes a great cup of coffee if you want to grab one."

Another situation in which location is important is when you find yourself being confronted by an unhappy physician. Unfortunately, physicians seldom choose the right place or time for these interactions. Use scripting to protect yourself. Say, "Dr. Thomas, I understand you're upset with me. Can we please go into my director's office and discuss this matter in private? I would like to have him hear what you have to say." If the director is not available, ask to have the supervisor paged and wait for his or her arrival.

## Scripting, in summation

Throughout this book, we've covered many areas and opportunities in which scripting can help you. From arriving at work to discussing a diagnosis with a physician, collaborating with peers, and discharging patients, scripting is a valuable skill to have in your nursing toolbox. It can help you out of a communication jam and can provide security in a tough conversation.

**Quick Highlight:** The secret to successful scripting is to make sure it doesn't sound, well, scripted. Using critical thinking and adapting to the conversation at hand will greatly improve your working environment.

As noted in Chapter 1, Wolfskill and Lipka affirm that scripting assists staff members in projecting the caring, professional image of the facility. We are all aware that, second only to patient safety, patient satisfaction is the top priority in healthcare today. Using skillfully drafted scripts, provided the user is sufficiently comfortable with doing so, can achieve both objectives.

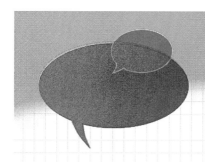

# References

Bloomfield, C. (2006). Scripting for success. *AORN Journal.* May 83(5): 1127–8

Davis, C. (2004). Breaking bad news. Retrieved April 1, 2009, from *www.medhunters.com/articles/breakingBadNews.html*

Do nurses have the time? (2009). Retrieved April 1, 2009, from *www.safestaffing.info/Do_Nurses_Have_The_Time_.html*

Get a high five for your patient care. (2009). Retrieved April 1, 2009, from *www.strategiesfornursemanagers.com/ce_detail/229137.cfm*

Govern, P. (2005). Service recovery initiatives outlined. Reporter: Vanderbilt Medical Center's Weekly Newspaper. Retrieved April 1, 2009, from *www.mc.vanderbilt.edu/reporter/index.html?ID=4176*

Hardwire the five fundamentals of service. The Studer Group. Retrieved April 1, 2009, from *www.studergroup.com/newsletter/Vol1_Issue3/ vol1_i3_sec7.htm*

How can nurse leaders boost patient satisfaction scores: An interview with Press Ganey's Deidra Mylod. Healthcare Financial Management Association. Retrieved April 1, 2009, from *www.hfma.org/publications/business_caring_newsletter/exclusives/How+Can+Nurse+Leaders+Boost+Patient+Satisfaction+Scores.htm*

Improving nurse-physician communication through the SBAR model. (2008). Robert Wood Johnson Foundation. Retrieved April 1, 2009, from *www.rwjf.org/pr/product.jsp?id=30312*

Lipka, M., & Wolfskill, S. (2008). *The Patient Access Director's Handbook.* Marblehead, MA: HCPro, Inc.

Miller, D. (2008). Improve patient safety and satisfaction through effective communication. *The Staff Educator*, an HCPro, Inc., publication 5(9): 5.

Mustard, L. (2003). Improving patient satisfaction through the consistent use of scripting by the nursing staff. *JONA'S Healthcare, Law, & Ethics* 5(3).

Navarro, J. (2008). What we say without words. *The Washington Post.* Retrieved March 18, 2009, from *www.washingtonpost.com/wpdyn/content/gallery/2008/06/23/GA2008062301669.html*

Newton-Wellesley RNs oppose Wal-Martization of nursing practice. (2006). *Massachusetts Nurse: The Newsletter of the Massachusetts Nurses Association.* Retrieved April 1, 2009, from *www.massnurses.org/files/file/News/newsletter/2006/April.pdf*

Ryan, J., & Wojciechowski, S. More than words ... Rx for scripting challenges: Best practice techniques. *Press Ganey Satisfaction Monitor* (2003).

Nonverbal communication. (2007). Retrieved March 27, 2009, from *www.fhsu. edu/~zhrepic/Teaching/GenEducation/nonverbcom/nonverbcom.htm*

Ramos, M. (2006). Eliminate destructive behaviors through example and evidence. *Nursing Management* 37(9): 34–41.

SBAR Toolkit. Arizona Hospital and Healthcare Association. Used with permission.

Scharf, A. (2003). Scripted talk: From "Welcome to McDonalds" to "Paper or plastic?" employers control the speech of service workers. *Dollars & Sense: The Magazine of Economic Justice.* Retrieved April 1, 2009, from *www.dollarsandsense.org/archives/2003/0903scharf.html*

Stevenson, K., Randle, J., & Grayling, I. (2006). Inter-group conflict in health care: UK students' experiences of bullying & the need for organizational solutions. *The Online Journal of Issues in Nursing.* Retrieved April 1, 2009, from *http://cms.nursingworld.org/MainMenuCategories/ANAMarketplace/ ANAPeriodicals/OJIN/TableofContents/Volume112006/No2May06/ tpc30_516077.aspx*

Yoder, E. (2007). Moving customer service scores with scripting and managing up techniques. *Radiology Management* 29(1): 50–3.

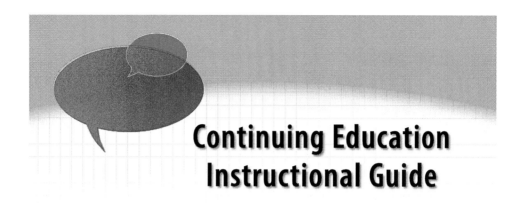

# Continuing Education Instructional Guide

## Quick-E! Pro Scripting: A Guide for Nurses

## Target Audience

Nurse managers

Staff development specialists

Directors of education

Staff educators

Staff nurses

## Statement of Need

With Centers for Medicare & Medicaid Services basing hospital reimbursement on patient satisfaction, giving nurses the tools they need to provide patients with quality care and information is essential. Nurses often don't get this information in nursing school and are pushed out into the working world with little idea of how to converse with patients, their families, or physicians. When they enter the work force, they are often timid and nervous about working with experienced physicians or difficult families. And when nurses don't interact positively with patients, satisfaction scores fall and safety is compromised. Our title will provide RNs with the confidence and know-how to communicate clearly and effectively.

## Educational Objectives

Upon completion of this activity, participants should be able to:

- Define scripting

- Identify two communication models often used in nursing

- List the components of SBAR

- Discuss the appropriate steps to take after a patient is admitted

- Identify a tool to use in helping assess a patient's pain

- Recognize the most effective time to give patients information about discharge

- List two actions that will make you more receptive to a patient when hearing a complaint

- List three items to have ready before calling a physician regarding a patient

- Identify two important items you should communicate to a peer in a shift report

- Discuss the "5 on the Board" program that improved patient satisfaction scores at CHRISTUS Hospital–St. Mary's in Port Arthur, TX

- Identify questions gathered by mystery shoppers that helped keep patient satisfaction scores high at CHRISTUS Hospital–St. Mary's

- List two additional ways to improve patient satisfaction scores

- Identify an appropriate comment to begin the process of delivering bad news to a patient

- Identify three of the most frequently reported negative behaviors by new nurses

- List two appropriate statements to make when you feel you are being ignored

- Choose one appropriate statement to make when thanking support personnel members for their help

- Identify how scripting can help with the HCAHPS hospital survey

- Explain how to use the mnemonic device "HEART" when discharging a patient

- Identify when scripting should not be used

## Faculty

**Kathleen L. Garrison, MSN, RN,** is the clinical educator in the training and development department at Prince William Hospital in Manassas, VA. She graduated in 1980 with her BSN from Fairfield (CT) University. She earned her master's degree in nursing in 2005 from George Mason University in Fairfax, VA.

**Jo-Ann C. Byrne, RN, BS, MHSA,** is the director of education and organizational development at St. Vincent's Healthcare in Jacksonville, FL, where she oversees all education, training development, and implementation activities for the hospital system.

**Frances Moore, RNC, BSN, MSA,** is manager of the department of education and organizational development at St. Vincent's HealthCare in Jacksonville, FL. She leads the education team for a two-hospital health system and is responsible for a variety of educational opportunities.

# Nursing Contact Hours

HCPro, Inc., is accredited as a provider of continuing nursing education by the American Nurses Credentialing Center Commission on Accreditation.

This educational activity for 3 nursing contact hours is provided by HCPro, Inc.

# Disclosure Statements

HCPro, Inc., has confirmed that none of the faculty or contributors have any relevant financial relationships to disclose related to the content of this educational activity.

# Instructions

To be eligible to receive your nursing contact hours or physician continuing education credits for this activity, you are required to do the following:

1.  Read the book *Quick-E! Pro Scripting: A Guide for Nurses*

2.  Complete the exam and receive a passing score of 80%

3.  Complete the evaluation

4.  Provide your contact information on the exam and evaluation

5.  Submit exam and evaluation to HCPro, Inc.

Please provide all of the information requested above and mail or fax your completed exam, program evaluation, and contact information to:

HCPro, Inc.

Attention: Continuing Education Manager

P.O. Box 1168

Marblehead, MA 01945

Fax: 781/639-2982

**NOTE:**

This book and associated exam are intended for individual use only. If you would like to provide this continuing education exam to other members of your nursing or physician staff, please contact our customer service department at 877/727-1728 to place your order. The exam fee schedule is as follows:

| Exam Quantity | Fee |
|---|---|
| 1 | $0 |
| 2–25 | $15 per person |
| 26–50 | $12 per person |
| 51–100 | $8 per person |
| 101+ | $5 per person |

## Continuing Education Exam

Name: _____

Title: _____

Facility name: _____

Address: _____

Address: _____

City: _____ State: _____ ZIP: _____

Phone number: _____ Fax number: _____

E-mail: _____

Date completed: _____

1.  **Scripting means:**

    a.  to follow a script

    b.  to say the same thing in every conversation

    c.  to provide carefully considered details as a plan of action

    d.  to answer in "yes" or "no" statements only

2.  **Which of the following is part of the acronym AIDET?**

    a.  Aware

    b.  Inspection

    c.  Ending

    d.  Thank you

3.  **Which of the following is part of the acronym SBAR?**

    a.  Situation

    b.  Backdrop

    c.  Addition

    d.  Recognition

**4.    The acronym SBAR is used for:**

    a.  nurse-physician interactions only

    b.  nurse-nurse interactions only

    c.  nurse-support staff interactions only

    d.  various communication between healthcare personnel

**5.    When orienting a patient to a room, it is important to focus on:**

    a.  doctor's orders

    b.  family services

    c.  bathroom location

    d.  activity level

**6.    What is the first step after a patient provides an answer based on the pain scale?**

    a.  Ensure the patient's comfort

    b.  Tell the patient you'll be back later

    c.  Introduce yourself

    d.  Establish an acceptable pain level

**7.    Why should you start discussing discharge plans with patients before their final day of care?**

    a.  It provides an opportunity for patients/families to learn more about their care process

    b.  They'll be more receptive to learning on their first day in the hospital

    c.  It gives all the nurses on the floor a chance to share their opinions

    d.  It gives support staff members a chance to share their opinions

8. **When listening to a patient complaint, be sure to:**

    a. stand while the patient is sitting to convey authority

    b. sit with a patient to let the patient know you're listening

    c. always pass the complaint on to your manager

    d. always include other nurses on the floor

9. **What should you make sure to do before calling a physician about a patient?**

    a. Confirm that the phone number is correct

    b. Sit in a comfortable chair

    c. Stand in the nurses' station

    d. Have either the test results or vital signs available

10. **When giving report to another nurse, be sure to mention the patient's:**

    a. living relatives

    b. occupation

    c. diet

    d. favorite physician

11. **What would managers and staff members at CHRISTUS Hospital–St. Mary's in Port Arthur, TX, do if a patient had a score lower than 5 on his or her white board?**

    a. Transfer the patient to another facility

    b. Have a staff meeting about the care at the facility

    c. Find out why and meet the patient's requests

    d. Ask physicians whether they can help with the patient

12. **Which of these questions did mystery shoppers at St. Mary's ask patients?**

    a. "How has your care been?"

    b. "Has your nurse visited you today?"

    c. "Do you know your manager's full name?"

    d. "Have you met your manager today?"

13. **Which of the following is a simple way to improve patient satisfaction scores?**

    a. Daily rounding

    b. Answering a call light in 30 seconds or less

    c. Answering a call light in 60 seconds or less

    d. Nurses and physicians rounding together

14. **If you are opening a conversation in which you have to convey unfortunate news to a patient, what would be an appropriate statement?**

    a. "You're not going to like this ..."

    b. "I'm sorry to have to tell you this ..."

    c. "The physician told me to tell you ..."

    d. " I'm in a hurry, so ..."

15. **According to a May 2006 study, being _____ is one of the most frequently reported negative behaviors experienced by new nurses.**

    a. criticized

    b. fired

    c. called in to work on weekends and holidays

    d. physically attacked

16. **Which of the following would be an appropriate statement to make if you feel you are being ignored?**

    a. "I hate when you guys don't include me."

    b. "I'm tired of not being included in everything."

    c. "Excuse me, I'd like to help."

    d. "You obviously don't need my help."

**17. When thanking support personnel members for their work, which of the following would be appropriate?**

    a. "I know you don't feel like you contribute, so I just wanted to say thanks."

    b. "Thank you for your extra effort today. You really made a difference."

    c. "You're really starting to pull your weight around here. Thanks."

    d. "Thanks for staying out of the way on this one."

**18. How can scripting be useful in preparation for the HCAHPS hospital survey?**

    a. Give patients a script to use when answering the questions

    b. Speak to patients using language they will recognize on the survey

    c. Hand patients some scripted questions and answers to make the process easier for them

    d. Instruct patients on how to fill out the survey

**19. In the mnemonic "HEART," which can be used when discharging patients, what does the "E" focus on?**

    a. Execution

    b. Energy

    c. Electronic

    d. Empathy

**20. It is unsafe to use scripting:**

    a. when communicating with peers

    b. when communicating with physicians

    c. when communicating with patients

    d. during emergencies

# Continuing Education Evaluation

Name: _____

Title: _____

Facility name: _____

Address: _____

Address: _____

City: _____ State: _____ ZIP: _____

Phone number: _____ Fax number: _____

E-mail: _____

Date completed: _____

1. **This activity met the learning objectives stated.**

   Strongly agree        Agree        Disagree        Strongly disagree

2. **Objectives were related to the overall purpose/goal of the activity.**

   Strongly agree        Agree        Disagree        Strongly disagree

3. **This activity was related to my continuing education needs.**

   Strongly agree        Agree        Disagree        Strongly disagree

4. **The exam for the activity was an accurate test of the knowledge gained.**

   Strongly agree        Agree        Disagree        Strongly disagree

5. **The activity avoided commercial bias or influence.**

   Strongly agree        Agree        Disagree        Strongly disagree

6. **This activity met my expectations.**

   Strongly agree          Agree          Disagree          Strongly disagree

7. **Will this activity enhance your professional practice?**

   Yes                   No

8. **The format was an appropriate method for delivery of the content for this activity.**

   Strongly agree          Agree          Disagree          Strongly disagree

9. **If you have any comments on this activity, please note them here:**

   _____

   _____

   _____

   _____

   _____

10. **How much time did it take for you to complete this activity?**

    _____

**Thank you for completing this evaluation of our continuing education activity!**

Return completed form to:

HCPro, Inc. • Attention: Continuing Education Manager

P.O. Box 1168, Marblehead, MA 01945 • Telephone: 877/727-1728 • Fax: 781/639-2982

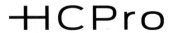